THE VITAMIN D CURE:

8 SURPRISING WAYS CURING YOUR UNDIAGNOSED VITAMIN D DEFICIENCY CAN REVITALIZE YOUR HEALTH, PREVENT CANCER AND HEART DISEASE, AND HELP YOU LOSE WEIGHT

BY RYAN J. S. MARTIN

First Printing: 2015

Bright Ideas Editorial

PO Box 4095

Crested Butte, CO 81224

https://www.facebook.com/brightideaseditoria

Disclaimer

Although the author and publisher have made every effort to ensure that the information in this book was correct at press time, the author and publisher do not assume and hereby disclaim any liability to any party for any loss, damage, or disruption caused by errors or omissions, whether such errors or omissions result from negligence, accident, or any other cause.

My Gift to You:

To download this free amazing book about powerful habits that can transform your body, mind, and spirit, go to
https://editoria.leadpages.net/25habits/ or my Facebook page.

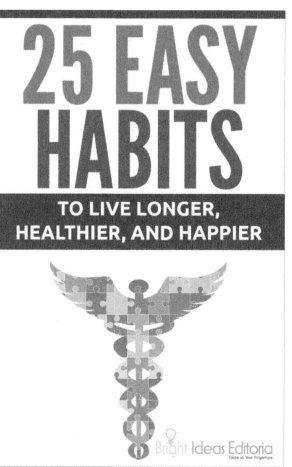

Table of Contents

Introduction

"For the sun, in rising and shining upon them purifies them."

HIPPOCRATES, FROM ON AIRS, WATERS AND PLACES

The Ancient Greeks, Egyptians, Romans, Assyrians, Chinese, and Incas all agreed that the sun had great power to regenerate the body. Though they might have each argued a different reason, they could demonstrate the sun's power to heal many conditions from diseases affecting the skin to those of the spirit. Today we know that the sun's restorative magic is the Vitamin D we absorb when UVB rays penetrate our skin. We also know that our evolved lifestyle means we do not get nearly enough of it.

If you live in the United States, there is somewhere between a 40% and 75% chance that you are not getting enough Vitamin D depending on which study you believe. Those odds rise steeply for African Americans, with some studies citing as high as a 90% deficiency rate among those with darker skin. The elderly, too, run an elevated risk. Moreover, this is not a uniquely American phenomenon. The latest numbers indicate that at least a billion people on the planet are suffering from moderate to severe Vitamin D deficiencies. Some are even calling it a pandemic. Diseases such as rickets that were thought to have been wiped out by supplementing milk in the 1930s are re-emerging in western nations.

The long Canadian winters mean that the majority of people in Canada are not getting enough D, particularly children. In Russia, China, and India, Vitamin D deficiencies among adults are quite high. So are levels across Europe.

But not everywhere. People who live in countries in Southeast Asia, including Thailand, have adequate Vitamin D levels, as do Australians and Japanese. Much of Africa appears to have escaped problems related to low Vitamin D levels, with the notable exception of South Africa.

Why is worldwide Vitamin D deficiency worthy of pandemic status? The Vitamin D Council in the United States links Vitamin D deficiency to no fewer than 45 different diseases and conditions, from acne to tuberculosis. Some of the more serious include diabetes, cancer, skeletal diseases, weakened immune systems, heart disease, sleep disorders, depression, and obesity.

Some countries are paying attention. In 2003, Finland increased Vitamin D food fortification and has since reported a number of benefits, including a drop in childhood type I diabetes. Other nations are looking carefully at their guidelines for supplements and fortifications. As these governments take action, researchers will have an easier time documenting cause and effect and advising which methods provide the most benefit.

In the meantime, it is up to individual doctors and patients to self-educate. Many doctors already include Vitamin D testing as part of their patient care. And many are not. Many patients who have a variety of symptoms from extreme fatigue to chronic muscle and bone pain are finding relief from a course of intense Vitamin D replenishment. And many remain undiagnosed, feeling helpless, unable to find relief.

This book seeks to understand what causes Vitamin D deficiency, explain how it can be diagnosed and treated, and to explore how adequate Vitamin D levels are essential for optimum health. Are you getting enough of the "miracle vitamin"? Can adding a Vitamin D supplement boost your health and improve the way you feel every day? Can it reduce your risk for a range of diseases, supercharge your immune system, strengthen your bones, and help you to lose weight? Take control of your body and begin feeling great as you participate in The Vitamin D Cure!

Chapter 1 – Understanding the Fundamentals of Vitamin D

Vitamin D was linked to strong bones in the early nineteenth century when doctors discovered that exposure to sunlight helped prevent rickets, a bone condition often found in children. In treating the condition, taking cod liver oil and basking in the sun helped considerably, and when milk was fortified wholesale with Vitamin D in western countries one hundred years later, the disease was nearly eradicated. The more researchers studied Vitamin D, the more it was found to be vital for overall health and not just bone health. In fact, Vitamin D can help prevent and treat some serious health issues.

Vitamin D is unique – quite unlike other vitamins that the body needs. In order to understand how it can do amazing things, we need to know exactly what Vitamin D is. Let's look at the basics of Vitamin D.

What is Vitamin D?

The most surprising fact about Vitamin D is that it is not even a vitamin. Not really. Medical experts say that it is more accurate to call it a hormone, because the body makes it on its own with a little help from the sun. Many other vitamins, like calcium, zinc, and potassium are elements you can point to on the periodic chart and they must be ingested.

Once the skin is exposed to the sun and Vitamin D is produced, it is sent to the liver for processing. When you swallow your Vitamin D supplement, the Vitamin D will also be sent to your liver through your digestive tract. Doctors call the substance that it is converted into "calcidiol" or 25(OH) D. This term is used to measure the amount of Vitamin D in the blood and refers to a serum.

It is this chemical that is transported all over the body to various tissues. It controls how much calcium is in the blood and bones, and in this way it aids the way all the cells in the body communicate. The kidneys will convert it into "activated Vitamin D," or calcitriol, and it can then go on into the body and perform a host of other functions. Vitamin D is a miracle vitamin, as it can be used by literally every cell in the body.

Types of Vitamin D: D2 vs D3

Vitamin D exists in two forms, Vitamin D3 and Vitamin D2. Vitamin D3 is produced in response to exposure to sunlight and is more common than Vitamin D2.

Vitamin D2 is also known as Ergocalciferol. It is not found on its own in nature; rather, it is derived from irradiated fungus. It is most likely to be found in fortified foods, especially cereals, plant foods and supplements. This Vitamin D is recommended by doctors if for any reason there is no Vitamin D3 available, and for vegetarians, but otherwise it is considered to be inferior.

Your body makes Vitamin D3, also known as Cholecalciferol, in the sun. It is also found in some fish. Vitamin D3 supplements are often made from the fat of lamb's wool or fish oil.

How is Vitamin D Useful for Overall Health?

Vitamin D improves the health and strength of your bones. It also helps increase the functionality of the heart, muscles, lungs and brain that help your body fight off a myriad of infections.

In bone development, calcium and phosphorus are vital for bone strength and structure development. Vitamin D is required for the absorption of these minerals. You can consume foods with adequate or even excess amounts of calcium and phosphorus, but without Vitamin D, your body will not be able to absorb these minerals.

Vitamin D has a range of benefits that it provides in the body and makes a significant difference to the health of bones, blood, and bodily organs. Vitamin D boosts various functions in the body including the prevention and treatment of:

Diabetes
Cancer
Skeletal diseases
Weakened immune systems
Heart and circulatory functionality
Sleep disorders
Depression
Obesity

Chapter 2: Where to Get Your Vitamin D

Vitamin D is distinctive compared to other vitamins because the body can create it on its own if it is exposed to direct sunlight. If you are not in a position to spend time in the sun, you can get Vitamin D from supplements. Vitamin D is present in trace amounts in a few foods, including oily fish, and in foods that have been fortified, like milk, yogurt, margarine, and cereal.

Exposing yourself to moderate amounts of sunlight can help with getting your daily dose of Vitamin D, although it might not be enough. This is especially true if you are unable to spend extended periods in the sun, or if due to weather conditions, you have no sunlight available at all. Unlike other vitamins, you cannot eat enough food to get your recommended dose of Vitamin D.

Vitamin D from sunlight comes from ultraviolet B (UVB) rays. The amount that your body can produce depends on various factors including:

What time of day you are exposed to the sun – The best rays of sunshine for Vitamin D absorption are those around midday. Early morning and late afternoon sunlight is inadequate because the atmosphere blocks out the valuable UVB rays at this time.

The country you live in – The closer the country you live in is to the equator, the easier it is for your skin to absorb Vitamin D. Areas which are far away from the equator experience extremes in their weather patterns, which will affect the amount of sunshine that is available.

Your skin color - People who have very pale skin do not need to spend a significant quantity of time in the sun for Vitamin D absorption. This is in direct contrast with those who have darker skins.

The amount you exercise – New research shows that people who regularly exercise have more 25 (OH) D in their blood. Particularly interesting is that this is found to be true whether or not the person is exercising outside.

Vitamin D and Sun Exposure

A good guideline as to when you have had enough is to be in the sun for half the time you need to be before you experience sunburn. A fair skinned person can be safely exposed for around 10 minutes, whereas a darker skinned person may need up to two hours of sun exposure. In this time, your body can produce between 10,000 and 25,000 IU of Vitamin D.

It is important that your skin is exposed in order for you to get any Vitamin D from the sun's rays, so going out in the sun wearing trousers and a long-sleeved shirt will limit how much Vitamin D your body can absorb. Ideally, any large surface area, such as your back, is optimal. It is not enough to try and get adequate Vitamin D by only exposing your face and arms.

Too much sun exposure, however, can lead to a sunburn. And sunburns can lead to skin cancer. Wearing sunblock is an excellent way to protect your skin from the sun's harmful rays, but it also blocks the beneficial ones. In fact, sunscreen can limit Vitamin D absorption by up to 95%. The arguably healthful habit of wearing sunblock when one is in the sun is a leading factor in the rise of Vitamin D deficiency. People are faced with walking a fine line to absorb enough sunlight to synthesize Vitamin D, but not so much as to burn.

There are other factors that affect how much Vitamin D your body can produce. The first of these is age. The older you are, the harder it becomes for your skin to produce Vitamin D. Therefore, older people are encouraged to take larger amounts of Vitamin D supplements.

On a cloudy day, your skin makes less Vitamin D, and this is also the case if you live somewhere there is excessive air pollution. This is simply because the sun's rays are blocked from reaching your skin. Also, the UVB rays do not pass through glass, so if you are in your car with the windows shut on a sunny day, your skin will not be able to produce Vitamin D.

Tanning beds can be an effective way to get your daily D if used correctly. Stick to short amounts of time, and make sure it is a low-pressure bed that has a good amount of UVB light.

Vitamin D in Food

The body makes its own Vitamin D by absorbing the sun's rays, and supplements also play an important role. However, there are some foods that contain small amounts of Vitamin D as well.

Vitamin D is present in cod liver oil, although so is Vitamin A – and in high doses. As both these vitamins are fat soluble, the body may face a challenge in absorbing the vitamin. Also, because the makeup of cod liver oil can vary widely depending on who manufactured it, doctors are now shying away from recommending it as a primary source for Vitamin D. Other foods that contain Vitamin D include fatty fish, like salmon and mackerel, fortified cereals, egg yolks, fortified milk and orange juice, beef liver and infant formula.

Once you know your recommended daily intake, you'll understand why most people rarely get all their Vitamin D from food alone. For example, a tablespoon full of cod liver oil contains 1260 IU of Vitamin D. A 3.5 ounce serving of cooked salmon has 360 IU of Vitamin D. The same amount of swordfish has even more, 566 IU, nearly a full day's worth for adults. Canned tuna has 154 IU per 3 ounces, and if you have a taste for sardines, they have 46 IU. Fortified milk contains 98 IU of Vitamin D per cup, one whole egg contains 20 IU, and fortified cereal contains 40 IU in each cup. Enriched yogurt can have up to 127 IU per cup. Beef liver and beef kidneys will give you around 40 IU per 3 ounces, but other red meats contain insignificant amounts.

Adults require a minimum of 600 IU of Vitamin D each day. They could conceivably get enough by eating cereal with milk for breakfast, a cup of fortified yogurt for lunch, and salmon for dinner, along with lots of fruits and veggies and perhaps whole grains to balance out the meals. But substitute chicken or meat for dinner, and suddenly the Vitamin D intake has been cut in half.

Chapter 3: Breaking Down Vitamin D Deficiency

I met a woman named Marianne in a Vitamin D discussion group, and I want to share her story with you. Marianne's legs hurt all the time. Over-the-counter pain medication helped little, and narcotic pain meds made her nauseous. Her doctor couldn't offer any explanation for her chronic pain, or for the persistent fatigue she was feeling. He suggested she look into taking up yoga and meditation in order to better balance the "stress" in her life. The forty-four-year-old administrator and mother of three had stress in spades, but she knew something else was going on. She guessed her symptoms were related to the weight she had put on over the years, or because perimenopause was beginning to set in, and she was frightened that things were never going to get better. Jeff, her husband, thought it was all in her head.

Finally, a friend convinced her to see a new doctor, who ordered a host of tests, including checking her Vitamin D. Marianne's levels were negligible. He placed her on a high dosage of weekly supplements, and after several months, she began to feel like herself again.

Marianne's story is extreme, but everyday people the world over complain to doctors about fatigue, muscle pain, depression, chronic illness, and more. And doctors are beginning to check Vitamin D levels more regularly. A 2009 study published in *The Scientific American* suggests that 75% of the US population is deficient in Vitamin D. The Center for Disease Control and Prevention says that number jumps up to 90% if you are African American. The good news is that this situation is expected to come under control in the coming years as doctors connect adding a daily supplement with mitigating or even curing a variety of symptoms.

Your body has a Vitamin D deficiency when it does not get enough Vitamin D for healthy functionality. If a child has a severe Vitamin D deficiency, they are said to have rickets. They could appear bow-legged and if they are very young, may even experience difficulty standing or moving around regularly. Sometimes the condition is mistaken for child abuse because the bones snap so easily.

When an adult has a severe Vitamin D deficiency, the condition is called osteomalacia. This deficiency can cause thin, soft, brittle bones, which could result in bone breaks due to falling or losing balance.

Vitamin D Deficiency has been linked to more serious health issues, some of which can be considered terminal. These include a range of cancers, high blood pressure, type II diabetes, asthma, type I diabetes, Alzheimer's and multiple sclerosis. Disorders that deal with the muscles may also occur as a result of Vitamin D deficiency.

Causes and Symptoms of Vitamin D Deficiency

The most likely causes of Vitamin D deficiency are:

The body is not exposed to enough sunlight. This is primarily because people spend a considerable amount of their time indoors. Another cause is the use of sunscreen that stops the skin from absorbing UVB rays.

Many people do not supplement adequately. Vitamin D is found in minor amounts in food; almost everyone inevitably has to take supplements, especially in the winter. If your body is severely deficient, the amount of D3 found in many popular multivitamins might not be enough.

Some people are more susceptible to Vitamin D deficiencies than others. These people include those with darker skin, especially black people. The more melanin there is in the skin, the harder it is to absorb the sun's rays. It has been found that people with very dark skin may have to have 25 times more exposure than those who are very fair.

Those who work indoors or in tunnels, in hospitals or through the night are also frequent victims as these people are unlikely to enjoy sun exposure. Also, people who cover their skin all the time, especially in colder places with fewer hours of sunlight each day. Older people who have thin skin may not be able to make adequate Vitamin D. And infants who are on exclusive breast milk, whose mothers do not take a supplement, and who are not exposed to the sun, are likely to have a deficiency. Pregnant women or the obese are also at risk as they need higher than average doses.

There are various symptoms that you can look out for to identify a severe Vitamin D deficiency. It is important to note that these symptoms are rather vague and in some cases, no symptoms may be present at all.

The symptoms include:
Tiredness
Aches and pains all over the body
Pain that feels like it is in the bones
General weakness in the body
Difficulty getting around and doing physical tasks
Frequent infections.

To check whether you have adequate Vitamin D in your body, doctors will take a blood test to check your 25(OH) D levels.

Consequences of Taking Too Much Vitamin D

Too much of a good thing can turn into something very bad. If you take Vitamin D supplements in excess, your body may end up with high levels of calcium developing in the blood. This leads to a condition known as hypercalcemia. The symptoms of this are:
Feelings of confusion
Exhaustion
Illness and thirst
Loss of appetite
Constant passing of urine
Weakness in the muscles and abdominal pain

To measure whether you have taken an excess of Vitamin D in supplements, the Doctor would need to carry out a blood test.

Vitamin D toxicity is also called Hypervitaminosis D, and it can be a potentially dangerous condition. It is often caused by taking mega doses of Vitamin supplements, rather than by excess exposure to the sun or from diet. The body has the ability to regulate how much Vitamin D it produces as a result of sun exposure, and foods just do not have enough Vitamin D to pose this type of risk (though eating excesses of foods rich in D can cause other problems).

Vitamin D toxicity causes calcium build up in the body, resulting in loss of appetite, nausea and other symptoms of hypercalcemia. Levels of toxicity are reached if more than 10,000 IU of Vitamin D are ingested each day for a period of several months.

There are several treatment options. The first is to stop taking Vitamin D in excess. Doctors may also prescribe corticosteroids or bisphosphonates and may also recommend that you lower the amount of calcium in the diet.

There are long-term complications that could come about as a result of Hypervitaminosis D if it is left untreated. These mainly have to do with the kidney, and they include kidney stones, kidney damage, and kidney failure. In addition, there could be excess bone loss causing calcification of the arteries and an increase in blood calcium that can cause abdominal heart rhythms.

Other than with a blood test, you could be diagnosed with Vitamin D toxicity following a urine test that checks for excess calcium or a bone x-ray looking for significant bone loss.

Serum Levels and Vitamin D – Understanding Lab Test Results

There is a global consensus that the serum level is the most important thing to note when checking on levels of Vitamin D in the body. This is what 25 (OH) D stands for. How the levels are interpreted, however, isn't quite as universally agreed upon, but the most common ranges used are as follows:

Level	25 (OH) D
Deficient	< 50 ng/ ml
Optimal	50 – 70 ng/ml
Treats cancer and heart disease	70 -100 ng/ml
Excess	> 100 ng/ml

Chapter 4: All You Need to Know About Vitamin D Supplements

It may be a challenge to spend enough time each day in sunlight in order to get the daily recommended intake of Vitamin D. Fortunately, supplements are readily available to help the body get what it needs.

There are two different types of Vitamin D supplements. The most highly recommended one is Vitamin D3. It is usually available as a tablet or capsule but is also available in some skin creams. The supplements are made from the fat of sheep wool or fish oil and are not vegetarian-friendly. Vitamin D3 mimics the functionality of Vitamin D that is created through sunlight.

Vitamin D2 supplements are plant based and are not as highly recommended, except for vegetarians. Vitamin D3 is converted more efficiently in the body, up to 500% faster than Vitamin D2. Vitamin D2 is also known to have a considerably shorter shelf life. Another disadvantage of Vitamin D2 is that its metabolites bind poorly with proteins, directly resulting in it being less effective than Vitamin D3.

Vitamin D supplements are available in a range of potencies, most commonly 5,000 IU or 10,000 IU per unit. For people who have very severe deficiencies, a doctor can prescribe a 50,000 IU dose to be taken once or twice a week only to avoid Vitamin D toxicity.

Vitamin D supplements are available as an emulsified oil drop, a chewable tablet, a capsule, or a topical cream. Some scientists believe that Vitamin D supplements are better absorbed if chewed and moved around under the tongue.

The Vitamin D supplement can be prescribed by a doctor, though many forms are available for purchase over the counter. It is important to check carefully on the dosage when buying these vitamins over the counter. The Vitamin D2 and Vitamin D3 supplements are usually the same price. There are currently Vitamin D3 supplements that also include calcium available on the market. These are often prescribed for people who have bone problems and need calcium, and better ensure that the calcium is absorbed as required.

For the best absorption results, Vitamin D supplements should be ingested with a meal that contains fat. If one takes a Vitamin D supplement on an empty stomach, the average rate of Vitamin D absorption decreases by 32%. The fat traveling together with the supplement means that the Vitamin D will not need to go through the body in order to find some fat beneath the skin.

Vitamin D supplements may interact with certain medications and be rendered ineffective. This is particularly true for steroid medications like Prednisone, which get in the way of Vitamin D metabolism. Before a person makes the decision to take over the counter Vitamin D, they should consult their doctor, especially if they are on any other type of medication.

In addition, certain weight loss drugs and seizure medications can also lead to issues with calcium absorption and Vitamin D metabolism. Drugs used for lowering cholesterol are known to increase the Vitamin D levels in the body. This sounds like a good thing, although it may dangerous if a supplement is also being taken at the same time.

Chapter 5: Recommended Guidelines for Vitamin D Intake

Around the globe, different organizations will provide their own recommendations of how much Vitamin D is required for a day. Some average figures for recommended minimum daily intakes are:

Age	Recommended Daily Intake
Infants	400 IU
Children	400 IU
Adults	600 IU
Seniors	800 IU

Between infants and adults, this dosage supports the notion that the bigger and heavier you get, the more Vitamin D that you need to ensure that your body can function at its maximum. Seniors need more Vitamin D as their thinner skin may make it more difficult for the sun's rays to be absorbed.

There are upper limits for these recommendations, particularly because some supplements are not available in smaller doses. Therefore one can take:

Age	Maximum Daily Intake
Infants	1000 – 1500 IU
Children	2500 - 3000 IU
Adults	4000 IU

The reason that it is important not to take in an excess amount of Vitamin D is that it is fat-soluble, meaning that any excess is stored in fat cells and can build up in the body over time. The upper limit for adults is 4000 IU each day, but that is taking into account that you spend some time in the sun. If you do not spend any time in the sun, some feel that you can take up to 10,000 IU a day, although you should check with a doctor. Anything above this is not considered safe or healthy. Repeated instances of Vitamin D overconsumption can lead to Vitamin D toxicity.

Vitamin D supplements are just that – supplements. It is still important to spend as much time in the sun as is possible and safe. Spending time in the sun is said to account for 10,000 – 25,000 IU of Vitamin D being produced in a day. The body knows how to regulate Vitamin D from the sun, which eliminates the issues of excess if only the sun is being used as a source.

Chapter 6: Vitamin D and Diabetes

Vitamin D has managed to pick up several nicknames over the years, including the 'sunshine vitamin' and the 'miracle vitamin'. Research has discovered that this Vitamin is excellent for the immune system, and some people have been bold enough to suggest that a healthy dose of Vitamin D is better than any vaccine.

This section shall explain the relationship between Vitamin D and some diseases, revealing how Vitamin D is an excellent choice for overall health and well-being.

Vitamin D and Type I Diabetes

Type I diabetes is an autoimmune disease, where the immune system attacks beta cells, the cells in the pancreas that help the body to produce the hormone known as insulin. Insulin assists the body in managing glucose, which turns food into energy for the body to use.

A link exists between type I diabetes and Vitamin D. Basically, it has been ascertained that those who had low Vitamin D intake in their first year of life were more susceptible to developing type I diabetes when they got older. Pregnant women deficient in Vitamin D can also affect their children, who might develop type I diabetes when they get older.

For the treatment of type I diabetes, taking Vitamin D supplements could help improve insulin sensitivity and aid the blood in controlling glucose levels. Although the research on the effectiveness of Vitamin D to treat type I diabetes is inconclusive, it is worth a try to improve health.

Vitamin D _**cannot**_ replace type I diabetes medication.

Vitamin D and Type II Diabetes

Type II diabetes is a condition where the body experiences difficulty when attempting to manage sugar correctly. It is often found in older adults and lasts for life.

If it is not adequately managed, a person can develop skin conditions, high blood pressure and problems with eyesight. This condition starts off as mild and gets worse with the passage of time. Towards the last stages of the condition, organ failure, infections on fingers and toes that lead to amputation, and urinary tract issues can occur.

Although research linking Vitamin D and type II diabetes is far from conclusive, there is one study which has found that younger people with high levels of Vitamin D in their systems are less likely to develop type II Diabetes in later life. This result was found when these people were directly compared with people who had lower levels of Vitamin D.

Taking a Vitamin D supplement when one is suffering from type II Diabetes has been found to help alleviate the symptoms. By no means is Vitamin D on its own a preventative solution for diabetes, however.

For the treatment of type II diabetes, Vitamin D has been found to help 'turn on' receptors in pancreatic beta cells that are not functioning correctly. This helps in the production of insulin. Vitamin D also helps significantly with the regulation of calcium. This is vital as calcium plays a role in controlling the release of insulin, which may affect beta cell functioning.

Chapter 7: Vitamin D and Cancer

There is a range of cancers that affect the body, and these cancers can attack any cell. They vary in their level of aggression and their locations, but they have one thing in common: if left completely untreated, they can result in death that comes before its time.

Vitamin D has been found to be of great help to cancer patients, as it helps with the symptoms. It can naturally assist to alleviate the mood, and can even help patients fight the disease when combined with other treatments. This chapter shall look at three common cancers and will explain how these cancers have been positively affected by Vitamin D.

Vitamin D and Colorectal Cancer

When a group of cancerous cells choose to grow in the rectum or colon, the resulting malignant tumor is referred to as colorectal cancer. To determine the stage of this cancer requires evaluating the size of the tumor, and whether it has spread to different parts of the body.

Research on this type of cancer and Vitamin D has unearthed that colorectal cancer patients are likely to have low levels of Vitamin D. In fact, people with higher levels of Vitamin D are less likely to develop colorectal cancer. For those who have already contracted this cancer, increasing their Vitamin D levels may cause a better overall outcome and help to prevent death from the cancer.

Vitamin D helps protect from colorectal cancer as it has receptors that are present on a cell's surface, where chemical signals are received. These receptors help the cell to behave in a particular way. Vitamin D can bind these receptors, causing signals to divide or die to not reach the cell and to avoid spreading around the body.

This research is mainly observational and should not be relied on entirely, especially if viewed as a substitute for medication.

Vitamin D and Breast Cancer

Breast cancer is caused by cancerous cells in and around the breast that result in a malignant tumor.

Women with breast cancer have been found to have reduced levels of Vitamin D in their systems. The likelihood of developing breast cancer decreases slightly among women who have higher levels of Vitamin D. For women who already have breast cancer, increasing their recommended daily levels of Vitamin D has revealed that their tumours can be smaller, and their chances of dying from breast cancer are reduced.

Vitamin D is not a treatment for breast cancer though it can help with getting healthier. It is important not to take an amount above the upper limit of the recommended daily intake. It is also important not to view taking Vitamin D as a replacement for other treatments.

Vitamin D works with breast cancer in the same way as it does with colorectal cancer – by binding the receptors that allow for chemical signals to be received.

Vitamin D and Prostate Cancer

Prostate cancer occurs when prostate cells, found in a small gland that is approximately the size of a walnut, grow abnormally resulting in clumps called tumors being formed. This cancer is particularly common in older men.

Vitamin D has been found to have a relationship with prostate cancer. Men with lower levels of Vitamin D are more susceptible to this cancer. Men who have this cancer but maintain healthy levels of Vitamin D are less likely to die from this cancer or to suffer from a particularly aggressive strain.

Like with the other cancers, Vitamin D attaches itself to the receptors on cells, causing delayed or stopped growth, death or reduced spread of the cancer cells.

Research is still being conducted on the effectiveness of Vitamin D and prostate cancer management. Vitamin D cannot be used as a replacement for treatment.

Chapter 8: Vitamin D and Other Conditions

In addition to cancer and diabetes, Vitamin D is of great assistance to the body when dealing with a range of other diseases. These diseases include those that are affected by problems with muscles and those that deal with the bone.

To further understand the effects that Vitamin D has on these diseases, this chapter elaborates on these issues.

Vitamin D and Skeletal Diseases

The core diseases that attack the bones are directly related to calcium and Vitamin D. When taking any dosage of calcium to be absorbed in the bones, it is important to take it with Vitamin D. This is because Vitamin D helps with calcium absorption, maintaining blood calcium levels, and prevention of very low blood calcium levels. Together with calcium, Vitamin D helps prevent bone diseases such as osteomalacia, osteoporosis, and osteopenia.

Older people suffering from skeletal diseases are at risk of enduring severe bone injuries in the event that they have a fall. Taking Vitamin D can prevent the 5.6% rate of fractures that occur in older people as a result of falling. Not only does Vitamin D strengthen the bones, but it also has receptors in muscle that improve muscle strength.

Strengthening muscles can also improve balance. In fact, research has found that supplementing 1000 IU per day of Vitamin D3 can reduce falls by up to 26%. Skeletal diseases due to a Vitamin D deficiency may also cause pain in the hips and knees. This can be corrected over time by increasing the levels of Vitamin D ingested on a daily basis.

Vitamin D and the Immune System

Scientists conducting research on Vitamin D have discovered that it has a role to play in strengthening the immune system. What is yet to be discovered is how much is needed to maximize the system.

This Vitamin is often called the 'miracle vitamin' because of what it can do within the body to promote overall health. Vitamin D is known to prevent autoimmunity. Autoimmunity occurs when cells in the immune system attack healthy cells in the body. Although it is not the only preventive measure for autoimmunity, the immune system does suffer when there is an absence of Vitamin D.

Vitamin D does this by avoiding triggering and arming T cells. T cells will attack the body's tissues when triggered through proteins, where the T-cell recognizes a native protein as foreign. This type of attack can eventually lead to the development of cancers, which could be terminal. For this reason, Vitamin D is said to help to prevent cancer.

As Vitamin D is vital for the health of the immune system, its presence helps to reduce the occurrence of many conditions, such as influenza. By building the immune system, even in the case of an outbreak, a person becomes less susceptible to getting the infection.

Vitamin D is said to increase the function of your immune system by a factor of 3 to 5. It also stimulates the production of the potent anti-microbial proteins. These are just what the body needs to fight off a large number of infections.

Vitamin D and Heart Disease

Research is now discovering that Vitamin D deficiency can lead to congestive heart failure, cardiovascular disease, peripheral arterial disease and heart attacks. Maintaining the minimum recommended daily intake is said to be a key to reducing the risk of heart disease.

Vitamin D can also lower the danger of developing heart disease as it helps lessen the occurrence of metabolic diseases such as diabetes and high blood pressure, decreasing inflammation, slowing down the thickening of the arterial walls and reducing the risk of arterial calcification or hardening.

A person who begins to take the recommended intake of Vitamin D while they are still young will significantly decrease the possibility of contracting heart disease as they get older.

Vitamin D and Pregnancy

Perhaps the most sensitive time in a woman's life is when she is pregnant and preparing to bring another human being into the world. It is at this time that most women will pay extra attention to their nutritional needs because they realize that there is someone else who is fully dependent on them for growth and development.

In order to help build up a developing baby's bones and teeth, the body needs Vitamin D to aid the absorption of calcium and phosphorus. In the case of any deficiency, the baby may have complications in life, including deformation of the skeleton or retardation of growth. This may be seen in low birth weight as well.

If a baby is born deficient in Vitamin D at birth, the baby is at higher risk of developing rickets. At such a young age, this may lead to deformity caused by fractures, as the bones are not strong enough to be protected from simple movements. In some cases, the physical development of the baby may be delayed. This deficiency can have a lifelong effect on the child's bone development and immune function.

For the expectant mom, a natural birth may be out of the question, as a deficiency of Vitamin D has been linked to preeclampsia that may cause early, emergency delivery of the baby through a caesarean section.

It is recommended that pregnant women consume 4000 IU of Vitamin D on a daily basis, especially if they are unable to spend time in direct sunlight. This amount should increase a little, possibly to 6000 IU per day, when they are lactating.

Women are often prescribed pre-natal supplements to make up for deficiencies in any vitamins when they are pregnant. However, these often do not contain an adequate amount of Vitamin

D, so an additional supplement, a Vitamin D rich diet, and exposure to sunlight are also highly recommended. Of course, a doctor should always be consulted before taking any supplements.

Vitamin D and Sleep

Parents often tell their children that they grow when they are asleep. The body is busy at work functioning in various ways, even when you are asleep. It is, therefore, no surprise that Vitamin D is needed by your body when you are sleeping and resting.

Many people suffer from sleep disorders of various kinds, and these disorders usually affect the quality of sleep. Some people are unable to fall asleep, some experience sleep apnea, and some sleep too much and so on. These disorders are often caused by insufficient nutrients in the system.

The intake of Vitamin D has been related to the body's ability to maintain a full night's sleep. The higher the intake of Vitamin D, the lower the risk of having problems with sleeping well.

Chapter 9: Vitamin D and Mental Health

Vitamin D is excellent when dealing with a range of physical illnesses and problem within the body, including those that affect body tissues and all the cells. In addition to all these physical illnesses, Vitamin D is also able to assist with mental illness so as to improve well-being, and lead to feeling great.

Primarily, Vitamin D has been linked with assisting with depression as detailed in this chapter.

Vitamin D and Depression

Unfortunately, the pressures of everyday life have led to increasing instances of depression all around the world. Depression is a mental disorder that affects one's mood. Today, depression is relatively common amongst people of all age groups and regardless of their social standing or background. People who are experiencing depression may feel sad, frustrated, and miserable for long durations of time.

If left untreated, depression and its symptoms can severely interfere with a person's day to day life, immobilizing them to the extent that they are unable to make any decisions, concentrate on anything or experience happiness in any form.

Vitamin D has an important part to play in mental health issues and their management. It has been found that Vitamin D can act on the parts of the brain that are linked to depression though more research needs to be done to determine exactly how this is possible.

There are various angles linking a lack of Vitamin D to an increase in occurrences of depression. The first link ties in with exposure to sunlight. Some people do suffer from depression because they do not spend enough time outdoors. However, researchers are still trying to agree on one point: whether a lack of Vitamin D causes depression or depression causes a lack of Vitamin D.

Vitamin D has a role to play chemically in combating depression. This ties in with how this Vitamin is excellent for the brain. Vitamin D helps to regulate adrenaline, noradrenaline and dopamine production in the brain. This is possible through Vitamin D receptors that can be found in the adrenal cortex. In addition Vitamin D offers protection against depletion of dopamine and serotonin. An 8-14% increase in depression has been associated with people who have a Vitamin D deficiency.

Researchers have also looked to establish a relationship between Vitamin D deficiency and suicide. It was discovered that lower levels of Vitamin D could increase the risk of suicide. The next stage of research intends to address whether increasing Vitamin D levels can have a positive effect on treatment for depression.

Vitamin D and Schizophrenia

In addition to depression, an absence or deficiency of Vitamin D has also been linked with another mental illness. Schizophrenia can occur in people who have abnormal amounts of Vitamin D in their systems. This is particularly true for newborn children whose birth mothers did not take an adequate amount of Vitamin D when they were pregnant. If the baby is born without schizophrenia, they are still at risk of developing the condition when they get older.

Chapter 10: Vitamin D and Weight

People who are overweight or obese have been found to be at greater risk of a Vitamin D deficiency. Even though increased sun exposure and a daily supplement (recommended dose) should help with the deficiency, it has been found that their bodies still end up short of what is required. It is, therefore, vital for a person who is overweight or obese to take a supplement to meet up with a deficiency. For these people, the potent Vitamin D3 supplements are recommended.

Obese people have problems releasing Vitamin D from the skin. This is believed to be because the fat round under the skin holds on to the vitamin, which is fat soluble.

There is also a gender element that affects Vitamin D and weight, especially when dealing with weight gain and weight loss. Women generally have more fat than men do, and, therefore, they experience slower release of Vitamin D from the skin as well. Therefore in women, some of the Vitamin D will travel to the liver for processing, whereas some will remain behind in the fat cells where the signal shall be sent for them to be stored.

Supplements can be taken on a daily, weekly or monthly basis. The amount that is to be taken is highly dependent on the dose that has been recommended by the doctor. If someone is simply looking to ensure they have all the nutrients in their body, they should take the smallest dose they can find, and ingest in once a day.

Anyone with a deficiency should check their Vitamin D levels every 2-3 months once they have started treatment. Taking in excess of the recommended upper limit Vitamin D can result in kidney and tissue damage. It can also cause a significant increase in haemoglobin AIC and C-reactive protein. The worst case scenario would be a rare case of Vitamin D toxicity.

Vitamin D and Weight Loss

There is research that supports the notion that Vitamin D may be good news for weight loss. It has been determined that every single type of cell in the body needs Vitamin D. This is even true for fat cells – which are the ones that most people are looking to get rid of when they start a weight loss diet plan.

Vitamin D is known for attaching itself to the receptors on cells, therefore influencing the messages or signals that these cells send out. The Vitamin D signal will communicate whether the body should burn fat or whether the fat should be stored. Typically, these receptors will indicate that fat should be burnt and the more they are burnt, they higher the chances of losing weight.

In addition, there are receptors found in the brain that help to control hunger pangs and cravings. Their receptors also help with alleviating one's mood, as they can increase the levels of the chemical serotonin. Vitamin D can send them the right signal, to control the desire to eat, and to avoid depression that may lead to emotional eating.

When it comes to Vitamin D assisting with weight loss, it optimizes the ability of the body to absorb nutrients that are important for weight loss, such as calcium. A body that is struggling with a lack of calcium (in case it is not properly absorbed) will likely have an increase of five times more than normal in the fatty acid synthase. This is bad news as it is enzymes in this acid that are known for converting calories into fat.

Introducing Vitamin D into the body can lead to a change to a fat burning state, rather than a fat storage state. This can actually speed up weight loss by up to 70%.

Chapter 11: Understanding Where Vitamin D Fits in the Paleo Diet

The Palo Diet has received an enormous amount of attention and has gained a huge and devoted following in recent years. The Paleo Diet is focused on getting healthier by eating the right foods, namely lean meats, vegetables, fruits, and nuts. It is not restrictive in regards to portions, and it does not require keeping track of all items that one eats or counting calories. It eliminates foods that are not in their original form, and that were not ingested during the Paleolithic period. The theory behind it is that over 10,000 years ago, our diet did not contain any processed or junk foods. Proponents believe that our bodies have not yet adapted to the changes in diet that have occurred since the Industrial Revolution, and we don't deal well with food that has been processed, or with grains or sugars.

The reason the diet is so popular is because many people have found they could change the way they eat, but still enjoy food, and lose weight at the same time.

One disadvantage to the Paleo Diet, though, is the lack of Vitamin D.

There is an imbalance of minerals and vitamins in this diet, where some are present in excess, and some are not present at all or are there in very low quantities. For example, the diet can provide a range of B vitamins due to the consumption of leafy vegetables, meat, and fish. There may be high levels of sodium from animal proteins. Calcium may be lacking in this diet because many people get their calcium from dairy products or fortified cereals. And it is hard on this diet to get enough Vitamin D. The foods that contain artificially fortified Vitamin D are often processed grains, cereals, and milk, which are not consumed in this diet.

Paleolithic man got plenty of Vitamin D because he spent a significant amount of time in the sun when hunting and gathering, and the human body can create Vitamin D following direct exposure to the sun. Things are different for people today. Modern lifestyles revolve around spending time in buildings or transportation vehicles, meaning that people will spend little or no time at all in the sun on a daily basis. Not spending time in the sun, and not consuming foods that are fortified with Vitamin D means that an individual on the Paleo Diet is likely to have a deficiency of this Vitamin.

As with any diet, it is important truly to understand all the different nutritional components that make up that diet. With the knowledge that this diet does not supply adequate Vitamin D, even with all its fresh food and vegetables, one can make a decision to take a supplement, in order to enable the body to operate at its maximum functionality.

Chapter 12: Vitamin D and Lifestyle

Now that Vitamin D is at the forefront, and there are numerous discussions and research projects underway to discover everything possible about it, it is important to try and repair the existing damage that has been done. This entails looking at reversing the issues with deficiency so that people can lead healthier lives. The best way to go about this it to address lifestyles, and how they can be changed or improved.

Inadequate Time Spent Outdoors in the Sunlight

Many people are experiencing Vitamin D deficiency because they are not spending enough time outdoors in the sun. This is best understood by considering an example of what the average person would do in a day.

When the average person starts their day, they may have a commute to their workplace, where they spend their time in a train, bus or car. They then spend the day working, often in front of a computer, from morning until evening. Even if they are able to open the windows at work, they will often be left shut to prevent wind from blowing away valuable papers.

At the end of the day, the person will leave work and commute back home, often as the sun is setting. This leaves no time during the day to spend in the sun. On weekends, this person might spend time lying in during the morning hours, and then catching up on household chores for the rest of the day. Again, no time is spent in the sun.

Perhaps this person will come alive at night, visiting a nightclub or going out for dinner to have a good time. Before one knows it, several months can go by without any time actually being spent in sunlight.

If this average person also has the added challenge of living in an area where there are long winters leading to even less sunshine than normal, then they are likely to have a Vitamin D deficiency.

This calls for a change of lifestyle in its entirety. The best sunlight for Vitamin D creation is that at midday. It is therefore encouraged for people to spend their lunch hour outdoors, enjoying the sunshine as they partake of the midday meal.

Also, people who live in areas where there is limited sunlight should take as much advantage as they can of the summer months. Light skinned individuals can commit to spending just 10 minutes a day to increase their Vitamin D levels, whereas, those with darker skin and the elderly can aim to spend half an hour each day in the sun.

During the months where there is limited sunshine, everyone should be encouraged to take supplements, on a daily basis, to meet the body's requirement for Vitamin D. This needs to be something that is viewed as routine, rather than as a special addition to an existing diet.

Consuming an Unbalanced Diet

What we put in our mouths to nourish our bodies plays a significant role in our overall health. By the increasing number of overweight and obese people all over the globe, it is a fact that much of the food being consumed is unhealthy.

Consumption of the wrong foods can lead to a range of diseases affecting the body. When these diseases occur, there is more strain or pressure on the body for Vitamin D, and if a person is not taking enough supplements to handle this pressure, then they add the problem of a Vitamin D deficiency.

It is time to change a lifestyle that revolves around convenience food, junk food, fried food and fast food, to one that is more thoughtful and healthy, to create a complete balance of vitamins, minerals and nutrients in the body.

There are diets that exist that attempt to do this, such as the Paleo Diet, but even these diets fall short when it comes to Vitamin

D. Whatever diet you may choose to be on, it is important that you are aware of all the sources of Vitamin D available, so that you know whether it is necessary to take supplements.

For a diet to have plenty of Vitamin D, it should include milk, eggs, liver, salmon and fortified cereals in generous amounts. Vegetables that have calcium should also be consumed, so that the Vitamin D can work with a mineral, which will prevent it from settling and taking root in a fat cell.

Although eating a diet that is full of Vitamin D-rich foods does not guarantee that it will possible to meet the minimum requirement each day, these foods can help to bridge a gap that could be caused by insufficient Vitamin D dosage from the sun or from a supplement.

Adopting a new lifestyle by spending more time outdoors and eating more Vitamin D rich foods shall go a long way in improving overall health. Awareness of your holistic diet is important to ensure you cover all nutritional bases.

Chapter 13: Amazing Tips on How Vitamin D Makes You Feel Great

This book has attempted to explain everything that you need to know about Vitamin D. This final chapter will touch on all the great things about Vitamin D, and how when you get the right amount, you can enjoy life more because you will be feeling great.

Enjoy Strong Bones – If you ever have the opportunity to speak with someone who is suffering from bone issues such as osteoporosis, you will have a new found appreciation for having strong bones. With strong bones you can safely participate in all sorts of physical activities, as well as experience improved balance, no pain in the joints and incredible posture. Vitamin D can help you experience this as your constant reality.

Helps maintain Healthy Hair – This is as a result of a spillover from other benefits. Vitamin D intake has been attributed to reducing stress levels. In addition, this means that there is also a decreased possibility of hair loss. Healthy hair has been found to contain Vitamin D in the follicles. Hair that is not healthy will not have any Vitamin D in its follicles.

Strengthen your Teeth – A big smile is an incredible gift to share with others, and it is even better if you have a beautiful set of teeth to show. Just as calcium is needed in the bones, it is also needed for teeth, and together with Vitamin D, strong teeth are the order of the day

Goes straight to your brain – Vitamin D helps brain functionality, which helps you stay sharp and alert, even as you get older. This can help you in every area of your life and in your interactions with other people. Imagine how rich your conversations can be when you can remember little details. Vitamin D is great in this regards.

Can help with all your cells – The cells in your body are meant to work like a machine to keep you going at full functionality. However, even machines need a little oil here and there to operate well. Vitamin D is that oil for your cells. By helping to nourish your cells, you enjoy the benefits of disease prevention and improved cell functionality. The plus side is that your mood can also change for the better, as you are likely to be calmer and happier.

Defense against Certain Diseases – Have you noticed that there is a flu going around? When you have a sufficient amount of Vitamin D in your system, you are less likely to catch the highly infectious flu. That is because your body is primed to fight off infections and even autoimmune diseases.

Prevents cancer – Vitamin D is known to help prevent some forms of cancer. Though this help is marginal in nature, the fact that it exists give people the opportunity to put up their best defense against the disease.

Conclusion

There is so much that Vitamin D can do in the body, and it is one vitamin that has been overlooked for a long time. All that has changed though, as more and more people are taking the time to understand how Vitamin D works within their bodies, and how it can improve their overall health, wellbeing, and happiness.

There are three places to get your Vitamin D, and that is from sunlight, through taking supplements and from the food that you consume.

For maximum Vitamin D production, a large area of skin, such as your back, should be exposed to the sun. Also, the closer to the equator you live, the easier it is for your body to produce Vitamin D. The sun's rays (UVB) are at the right angle for absorption close to midday, so that is when you should expose your skin.

The amount of melanin in your skin will affect absorption of UVB rays.

Should you choose to get your Vitamin D from supplements, you should note the dose that you are taking. There are negatives that occur if you take a dose that is too low, or if you go overboard and take a dose that is too high.

Although Vitamin D can also be found in a few foods, the amounts in these foods is rarely enough to meet the required recommended daily intake, therefore, one must also spend time in the sun or take a supplement.

It is excellent that Vitamin D is getting more and more recognition nowadays because it has a role to play in improving the immune system and fighting disease. Many people are making the wrong lifestyle choices, and the result of that is a sharp increase in the number of people who are suffering from terminal diseases.

Vitamin D may not be a cure, but it offers preventive hope, as well as helping to manage the symptoms of a range of diseases.

Vitamin D is also excellent for people suffering from mental health issues, as it is known to go into the brain and help control all the receptors that are sending signals to take certain actions. It promotes better brain functionality that can reduce stress levels considerably and increase the levels of happiness.

Finally, Vitamin D is also excellent for people who are attempting to lose weight. It helps other nutrients in the body work efficiently, making it easier for the body to break down fat, which eventually leads to weight loss.

This book intended to provide you with a holistic view of Vitamin D – what it does for the body, the consequences of a deficiency or having it in excess, its power in fighting diseases and its ability to make life happier. Make sure that you are taking your recommended daily dose, and watch the transformation that will occur in your health, and in your life.

Message from the Author

One of the reasons that I love researching and writing in the information age is that it is easier than ever to connect with readers. Many of you generously let me know about new data and studies when they first come available, and even share with me your own personal stories. Please keep your comments coming. You can connect with me by email at ryanjsmartin@gmail.com, via twitter at @ryanjsmartin, or on my Facebook page.

If you'd like to help other readers decide if this book is for them, I'd be grateful if you could take a moment and post a sentence or two as a review. Reader comments are the most powerful and unbiased way for others to determine which books should make the short list for their next read.

If you're looking for more information about preventing and treating illnesses with vitamins and minerals, take a look at my latest book, *Magnesium Deficiency*.

To your health,

Ryan

Additional Resources

Association, A. P., 2014. *VItamin D and Pregnancy.* [Online]
Available at: http://americanpregnancy.org/pregnancy-health/vitamin-d-and-pregnancy/
[Accessed March 25 2015].

Bembu, 2015. *17 Benefits of Vitamin D for Your Health & Wellness.*
[Online]
Available at: http://bembu.com/vitamin-d-benefits
[Accessed 25 March 2015].

Choices, N., 2013. *How to get Vitamin D from Sunligt.* [Online]
Available at: http://www.nhs.uk/Livewell/Summerhealth/Pages/vitamin-D-sunlight.aspx
[Accessed 26 March 2015].

Clinic, C., 2015. *Vitamin D and Heart Disease.* [Online]
Available at:
http://my.clevelandclinic.org/services/heart/prevention/emotional-health/holistic-therapies/vitamin-d-heart-disease
[Accessed 24 March 2015].

Clinic, M., 2015. *Vitamin D Drugs and Supplements.* [Online]
Available at: http://www.mayoclinic.org/drugs-supplements/vitamin-d/evidence/hrb-20060400
[Accessed 24 March 2015].

Council, V. D., 2015. *Influenza.* [Online]
Available at: https://www.vitamindcouncil.org/health-conditions/influenza/
[Accessed 24 March 2015].

Council, V. D., 2015. *Vitamin D may relate to a specific sleep symptom.*
[Online]
Available at: https://www.vitamindcouncil.org/vitamin-d-news/vitamin-d-may-relate-to-a-specific-sleep-symptom-says-new-study/
[Accessed 25 March 2015].

Council, V. D., 2015. *What is Vitamin D.* [Online]
Available at: https://www.vitamindcouncil.org/about-vitamin-d/what-is-vitamin-d/
[Accessed 26 March 2015].

Hiatt, K., 2015. *Paleo Diet.* [Online]
Available at: http://health.usnews.com/best-diet/paleo-diet
[Accessed 19 March 2015].

Hutch, F., 2014. *Vitamin D and its effect on weight loss examined in new study.* [Online]
Available at:
https://www.fredhutch.org/en/news/releases/2014/04/vitamin-d-effect-on-weight-loss.html
[Accessed 23 March 2015].

Mercola, 2012. *Why Vitamin D Is Better than ANY Vaccine and Improves Your Immune System by 3-5 Times.* [Online]
Available at:
http://articles.mercola.com/sites/articles/archive/2012/01/04/why-this-vitamin-is-better-than-any-vaccine-and-improves-your-immune-system-by-35-times.aspx
[Accessed 26 March 2015].

PaleoLeap, 2014. *Everything You Need to Know About Vitamin D.* [Online]
Available at: http://paleoleap.com/vitamin-d/
[Accessed 19 March 2015].

Printed in Great Britain
by Amazon

36337358R00031